Medical Receptionist
Handbook to Success

Medical Receptionist Handbook to Success

Copyright © 2018 by Shivhon Adkins

All Rights Reserved

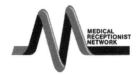

Medical Receptionist Network

ISBN: 978-0692066867

Book cover and book interior by Jean Boles
https://www.upwork.com/fl/jeanboles

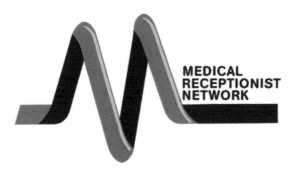

Medical Receptionist
Handbook to Success

Created for Medical Receptionists,
Medical Secretaries and Unit Secretaries
who are making a difference in the
healthcare industry

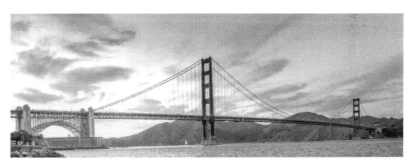

You are the BRIDGE!

Shivhon Adkins

Join the Medical Receptionist Network Community

Are you Medical Receptionist Network Certified? Visit our site to get started: www.medicalreceptionistnetwork.com

Join the conversation: MRN Podcast:
https://mrn.podbean.com/

Follow Us on Social Media

Like our Facebook Page
https://www.facebook.com/medicalreceptionistnetwork

Join our Facebook Group
https://www.facebook.com/groups/medicalreceptionistnetwork/

Follow Us on Twitter
@ReceptionistNet
https://twitter.com/ReceptionistNet

CONTENTS

PREFACE

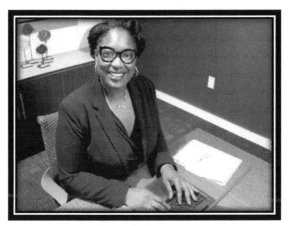

Shivhon Adkins

As a former medical receptionist and also the manager of medical receptionists, I truly understand the importance of this extraordinary role in healthcare. I remember starting my first position in an urgent care center, working behind a small desk with two or three other receptionists and our supervisor. It was in a fast-paced environment and I had no idea what I was doing. That changed quickly. While I thought I was learning how to check in patients, complete referrals, and answer and respond to countless phone calls, I was also learning the vital skills I needed to move forward in my career and in my life.

When you deal with different people from all walks of life and from various countries, who speak various languages, and are suffering from a multitude of ailments and present with different needs, you will learn a lot. When you work side by side with coworkers who have different backgrounds, different skill sets, and different attitudes, you will learn a lot. When you can work with physicians and other healthcare practitioners who have different styles of practice, different expectations, and high standards, you learn a lot. When you are advised by managers, administrators, and supervisors who want the patients to have a great experience, who want all policies and procedures followed, and who don't always have the answers but are willing to figure things out, you learn a lot.

It took me many years to truly understand the value of the experiences I had while I was a medical receptionist. I received positive feedback during those years; I learned new skills; I trained others, and I had patients that were "my patients" because they knew if they called for me, their request would be handled appropriately. I even received an Outstanding Employee Award because "nothing ruffled my feathers." This didn't happen because I am special or because I have a high IQ, and I didn't think I was better than those who worked alongside of me. My experience was positive because I paid attention; I was open to learning, open to helping, willing to spend that extra minute with a patient, willing to accept constructive criticism, willing to pick up the phone on the first ring. Most importantly, I knew when to ask for assistance and present a positive attitude no matter how I was feeling or how the person on the other end of the desk was presenting themselves at that moment.

When you are employed by anyone, you are an agent on behalf of that company, that practice, that hospital or care center.

Medical Receptionists work in so many different settings—from internal medicine, pediatrics, mental health, obstetrics and gynecology, neurology, dentistry, oncology, veterinary and substance abuse clinics, just to name a few. There are unit secretaries working in hospitals and nursing homes, providing support to nursing staff and physicians.

Your role in healthcare is a bridge: a bridge of communication between doctor and patient, between labs and nurses, between specialists and Primary Care Physicians, between insurance companies and billers, between drug representatives and practitioners. People must communicate with you to move through the process. **You are the bridge**. I want to help you be the strongest bridge you can be. This handbook will serve as your guide; it will serve as a reminder of how your ability can strengthen your workplace if you embrace it. Your time and effort are valuable and your support is needed. Ladies and gentlemen, please enjoy this handbook that I have created with only YOU in mind.

ACKNOWLEDGEMENTS

I must first thank you, Mom, for always supporting my journey in and outside of healthcare. Your career as a nurse allowed me to see what true compassion and dedication was all about. Your encouragement throughout my own career and the empowering conversations we shared allowed me to come as far as I have today.

To all my past managers, from supervisors to physician owners, I appreciate you giving me the chance to shine and not stifle my aspirations and abilities. Growth is essential, and I was able to do that.

To my past coworkers, thank you for showing me the way when I needed it and thank you for allowing me to show you the way when you needed it.

As a manager I thank and appreciate my past employees for allowing me to lead genuinely and fairly, for listening, for being honest, and for being my rock when we had so much coming at us at once. I hope you can say as much for me. It was always a pleasure.

Special thanks to Edison Emergi Med, the physician leaders of Brunswick Hills Obstetrics and Gynecology, Balancing Health, and Advocare Newborn Network.

Finally, I want to thank my family and friends for all of their support and cheerleading along the way!   ′

Medical Receptionist Network is a pathway to share the experiences of my career in order to encourage, provide training, and empowerment to Medical Receptionists nationwide.

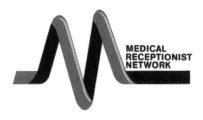

INTRODUCTION

Healthcare has created millions of jobs. There are so many options and avenues to enter the healthcare industry, and many of them do not require you to have a PhD. Providing services in the role of a Medical Receptionist is one of those avenues. You have a front row seat to this industry. You are providing and collecting information and providing administrative and clerical support. You are receiving a great deal of information which is often private and protected. You have a responsibility to always be courteous and respectful to your patients while assisting and guiding them through any process required by your office, hospital or healthcare organization.

When a patient, family member or friend walk into your healthcare facility, nine times out of ten, you are the first person they encounter, you are the initial point of contact, you are the first source of information, and you will be the first impression of your organization. To me, that sounds like a huge responsibility, and all of that happens in the first few minutes or even seconds!

Time is valuable, and everyone's time serves different purposes. When you are at work, your time should be spent by being fully present, aware and interactive in order to execute all of your tasks efficiently. The patients' time is spent making sure they have filled out all the right forms, that they have all the right documents, test results, and payment. They may also be concerned about getting back to work, or anxious because they are in the office to obtain some important results, or maybe they hate needles, and suffer from "white coat syndrome" and are trying to do all their paperwork with a rising blood pressure that was fine before they walked in.

You are probably wondering how YOU being fully present is going to help any of this. Well listen, if you are using your time wisely and taking the steps required to update paperwork, scan cards, call for reports, and pay attention to the people, to the patients who are interacting with you, you will begin to sense when people need extra help. You will actually notice when someone is in distress; you will notice when someone needs help reading or writing. You will learn when and how to move between a phone call and the person standing in front of you. It all has to do with time and action. Not reaction!

In this handbook, you will learn what attributes are a must when it comes to being a fantastic Medical Receptionist, Unit Secretary, and other clerical roles in healthcare. Take every situation or any scenario that comes your way and learn from it.

Don't fight it, don't lash out, and don't become discouraged. You are the bridge, and that is a very important job!

BEST PRACTICES

Customer Service

Customer service is the #1 responsibility of any Medical Receptionist. This term is tossed around all the time; let's dig deeper to highlight why it is a part of your best practices. The Business Dictionary defines Customer Service as *All interactions between a customer and a product provider at the time of sale, and thereafter. Customer service adds value to a product and builds enduring relationships.*[1]

You may be saying to yourself, "I am not selling anything." "We don't have products." Perhaps this definition will resonate more: *All interactions between a patient and our services and providers at time of service, and thereafter. Customer service adds value to our organization and builds enduring relationships.*

Providing good customer service in healthcare is more than just being polite and flashing a smile. You are

---

[1] http://www.businessdictionary.com/definition/customer-service.html

required to be courteous, observant, knowledgeable, self-sufficient, timely, responsive, responsible, understanding, and reliable. While this may not be stated word for word in your job description, it is most definitely expected. Providing good customer service to patients requires that you make sure the people you encounter day in and day out are satisfied. You are probably thinking, "I can't make everyone happy!" I didn't say "happy," I said satisfied.

What falls under "satisfaction" for a patient in an office setting?

Acknowledge, Action, Assist, Explain!

Acknowledge - Don't ignore people when they walk in, use your voice, your hand, a great big smile to acknowledge their presence. This is especially important at the front desk.

Action - Be attentive during your communication. If the patient has a question, look up and away from the computer when you respond. If they need immediate medical attention get them help! I am not saying you should be running around the office. I am saying if you act, the patient feels acknowledged! "Wow, she really wanted to make sure my questions were answered." or "I'm glad he quickly got the nurse or the wheelchair before I passed out." Those sound like phrases of someone who is SATISFIED with the level of service they received.

Assist and Explain - Sometimes people won't always ask for help. If you notice someone taking longer than usual to complete forms, ask if there is anything you can help them with. If they question a policy or medical procedure, explain it or get someone who can! The last thing you want is people walking out of your office completely confused. This tends to happen when people are checking out or leaving a medical facility. Lastly, before you ever say "NO" to a patient, you must be clear on what they are asking and have an explanation or reason to support your answer. If you don't know why your office doesn't do something, or when they stopped taking a certain insurance—guess what? You should! You are the bridge. Engage with your manager or administrator and keep notes on most common questions.

Acknowledge, Take Action, Assist, and Explain!

Knowledge

Knowledge is the next best practice we will discuss. As a medical receptionist, medical secretary or unit secretary, it is your responsibility to know about the healthcare center or medical office you work for. Knowing as much as you can will build your confidence in your position and show that you are serious about your role in the organization. Knowledge as defined by the Merriam Webster dictionary[2] as

- the fact or condition of knowing something with familiarity gained through experience or association

- the fact or condition of being aware of something: the range of one's information or understanding

YOU are a provider of information and that requires that you understand and are aware of the information that is specific to your patients. One of the first things you should do when starting a new job is take a tour. Make sure you know where things are or how to get them, who you can get them from, and how you need to request certain supplies or other office items. During training you will learn a ton of information—will you remember everything on day one? Of course not, but you should take notes. I have realized over the years that everyone does not find note taking beneficial while training; however, if you find a process is more difficult, lengthy or will require you to ask more questions, take

---

[2] https://www.merriam-webster.com/dictionary/knowledge

those notes and review them for a few nights. If you don't, you will be asking your co-workers the SAME questions repeatedly. I have seen it happen—the person asking the question has not a single note to refer to.

Lack of knowledge of your job functions can cause you to be in a position where you are inefficient, you may become a distraction to co-workers, and you will not build the self-esteem required for you to excel! I want you to succeed; you must have the knowledge and tools to be exceptional.

Once you get beyond the point of basic training it is important that you take the steps to understand what each appointment entails at your practice or organization. Understand the estimated time and allotted appointment times. Be knowledgeable of the procedures performed in your office.

For instance, if you have a patient who has all the paperwork for surgery and you know from prior experience that the information about driving post-surgery is included, on the way out the patient asks, *"When will I be able to drive after surgery?"*

Response 1: *"I don't know, but it is in your packet. I suggest you read it."*

Or,

> **Response 2:** "*Typically patients can begin driving after their first post-operative appointment. I do recommend that you review your surgery packet tonight. We have included all of that information for you.*"

If you use the second response, the patient has been provided an answer and redirected to the importance of reading the packet. You did that without giving any medical information or a direct order. You are reinforcing that the information the physician or nurse gave the patient is important. If you did not know what was included in the packet, you would not be able to confidently answer that question. Think of an example that would fit your practice. Is there a question you would like to be more equipped to answer, or information that you need readily available to you but have never sought it out or requested it from your employer? Write it down so you won't forget.

_____

_____

_____

_____

_____

_____

Most practices have pamphlets about office procedures, surgeries, vaccines, and programs/classes your office may offer. You should have read them all! You should not just know what something is called; you should be able to explain, or at least describe it, to another person. The information is in your face every day. It is FREE to read! While you may feel it is not necessary for your current position, why would you deprive yourself of the knowledge, deprive yourself of the ability to engage with your patients and providers about the medical care that is provided in the office. If you work in a specialist office and then move to Family Practice and maybe a few years later you decide you want to work in a surgical center—YOU will have to learn something new every time—get used to it! Every office is different, but being knowledgeable about the on-goings while you are a part of the team makes you a true asset.

Communication

Communication is the third best practice that we will discuss. We have focused a lot on patient care and the quality that you bring when you provide and combine great customer service and are knowledgeable about the area of health care you are active in. Now it's time to focus on how you are communicating with everyone. This includes patients, providers, coworkers, managers, pharmaceutical representatives, and other business partners.

Communication[3] is defined as:

- a process by which information is exchanged between individuals through a common system of symbols, signs, or behavior

- exchange of information

- a verbal or written message

Communication is more than just words. If you were to have a disagreement with your coworker and you did not resolve the issue right away, tension may be present. How would that come across to the patient walking up to the desk or to a caller on the phone, or even another coworker when they come to ask if you want to order lunch. Your tension can be felt in your tone of voice, your body language, or your attitude. You are communicating in a manner that is not open, and you are not ready to receive or to be fully present in the moment that is in no way connected to the disagreement you participated in. Avoiding these reactions is really a part of being professional. The way

---

[3] https://www.merriam-webster.com/dictionary/communication?src=search-dict-box

you communicate can cause a reaction or domino effect, but only if you allow it!

It's time to discuss communication with your manager, practice administrator, clinical staff, and other co-workers within your medical office or organization.

A well-oiled machine doesn't run with a few good parts and parts that often break and fall apart. A well-oiled machine requires all good and fully functioning parts! The people you work with are part of the machine; having meaningful and effective communication with them is extremely important. Don't hold back vital information; if the patient asks you to "take a note" or "please tell the doctor," don't make assumptions. Do not assume that the patient will tell the doctor again when they see them, don't assume that they will request that refill when they see the nurse, don't assume that they will call back to request a referral. If the patient felt the need to inform you, it is most likely because they believe you will handle the request.

Why not create a phone note or add a note into your Electronic Medical Record system? You can even write it down and hand to the provider or the nurse or medical assistant that will be helping the patient. Don't misunderstand me, if a patient is inquiring about clinical information, always redirect to the nurse or physician who can provide an answer to avoid liability of false or incorrect information.

Communicating with management and providers can be intimidating or scary for some. They may have more education or even more experience than you, or vice versa, but those things have nothing to do with how anyone is treated in the workplace. Communication is a two-way street! You should always make sure that you are clearly communicating with your management and providers regarding patients or your own needs and requests. Always use modes of communication that are acceptable within your setting: phone calls, meetings, email, text, and/or inter-office messaging.

When you use proper protocol to start you have a better chance of resolution or results. You must not let issues fester, whether it be related to the computer systems, your vacation time, or your co-workers. The earlier you tackle concerns the less significant their impact will be. If you have an issue with how someone communicates with you, make sure you address it and seek out solutions to improve so the issue does not affect the morale or effectiveness of your organization. Be clear and always take notes so you don't get rushed away without making your point and having your voice heard.

You have a right to communicate with the providers about their patients; you have a right to request a meeting with your manager to discuss your position and responsibilities. Do not wait for people to acknowledge you. You are part of a team. Imagine going weeks without certain parts of your team. Have you ever experienced the sudden absence of a team member? How did it affect your daily operations?

_____

_____

_____

_____

_____

_____

_____

_____

_____

_____

_____

LEVEL UP

Now that you understand the basics of **Customer Service, Knowledge** of the workplace and **Communication**, it's time to level up! How do you become the most skilled medical receptionist, medical secretary, or unit secretary? I have found that the skills and abilities required to start your career do not usually require a college education. There are skills that you can learn in or outside of a traditional classroom that will make you stand out, become more valuable to your employer, boost your confidence and self-esteem, and eventually, your salary or wages.

More than 80% of medical practices are using Electronic Health Record Systems. I will not assume that everyone is computer savvy because even in this day and age some people do not use computers, smartphones, and tablets as much as we may think. Healthcare has changed, and the technology has advanced with it. Having basic knowledge of how to use a computer is a must. Being able to type at a moderate speed is also required. Even if an office or hospital is not yet fully integrated with EHR and Patient Management (PM) systems, you will still want to have these skills under your belt. If you are just starting out, there are plenty of free resources online to help with basic programs like Word and Excel and even help you to improve your typing speed. An understanding of Microsoft Office is important because many EHR/EMR systems create letters and patient communication documents through Word. You may be responsible for editing and creation of letters in your role as a medical receptionist.

Taking messages and making appointments is also done using the EHR or EMR system. On-the-job training will help you navigate the system, but the basic knowledge of knowing how to shut down your computer, restart, where to find the print function, using ctrl, tab, and shift keys should really be known before you walk through the door. Your personality will not hide the fact that you did not take the time to learn anything on your own! You must *level up*, no matter where you are with your skills. When you change jobs or get an offer, you can inquire about what system is used in the office or the facility. There are many YouTube videos and demos online. You can at least see what the system looks like and how it operates before your first day of work. YOU will feel more prepared and confident and your employer will take notice of your eagerness to learn.

Basic computer skills are not the only way to *level up.* You will deal with people every day so you should know how to approach situations with an open mind and respectful manner. Why not take a course on communication in healthcare or medical terminology? Understanding healthcare privacy and employee rights will keep you on top of your game. Don't rely on someone else to give you information when you can access it yourself.

PROFESSIONALISM

Be a Pro. Once you have the knowledge, the communication, and the resources, you should dominate your space. Don't allow your location, salary, or the actions and opinions of your colleagues to affect how you operate daily. Be on time and show up ready to work, ready to serve your patients/clients. Do not be the first person in the office to make a negative comment about the day or about your personal life. When people set those standards, they must live in them. If you are rude to the people around you it creates an uninviting environment. Since you must spend so much time there, why not do your part in keeping things flowing and be as positive as possible.

When someone calls on the phone, they can't see how busy you may be, and they don't need to hear it in your voice. When the tables are turned, and a provider or member of the management team projects their negative feelings or thoughts to you, how do you feel? Probably not great. It works in every direction, including with patients. If people approach you and they are negative and you respond on that same level, nothing is accomplished. Do not allow others to change your mind about how you are feeling.

What else contributes to being professional? **How you dress, hygiene, teamwork, taking responsibility, continued growth.** Let's dive in. Professional dress doesn't mean expensive; however, it does mean clean, pressed and suitable for the work environment. That may be business casual or scrubs—scrubs which should not look like you grabbed them out of the laundry basket or off the floor. I've seen it time and time again. It's obvious and it is sloppy. You are the representative for an organization and for yourself; it is important to follow through in all areas. If your body odor or breath is offensive, people won't want to communicate with you as freely, and that is not productive. It's a stop sign or at least a yellow caution light of communication.

Hygiene is huge and bad hygiene affects others if not taken seriously. Most medical offices and healthcare facilities become very busy throughout the day. You may even break a sweat. Deodorant and clean clothes will help you from becoming offensive. Don't try to cover up with perfume; strong perfume can cause certain people to have a reaction, including allergy related or headache. Brushing your teeth and daily showers are also required. Some of you reading this are saying, "Really?!" Yes, really. Not everyone practices the same daily habits and do not find the same things "normal" or general knowledge. It is important to think of this when you encounter someone who may be offensive in your office or practice. Managers and administrators deal with this issue frequently. Often it goes unresolved because everyone is tiptoeing around the issue, hoping the person will change their ways. That is where communication comes in! I am not saying it is your responsibility to deal with the person directly but at least notify a manager or supervisor who will. While you may have a great working relationship with someone, that doesn't mean that you telling them that they smell is going to go over well. Being direct and speaking in private often makes these types of situations more bearable and resolvable for staff and management!

Next, we have the teamwork aspect of being a pro. Being part of a team is great—listening to others, sharing ideas, having the same appreciation for your employer and patients, making every day the best it could be. Always think of yourself as a leader. Don't try to be the "boss," even if you are the most experienced. Be a leader and lead by example. Assist others. When someone needs help with a process, don't take over, show them how or send them on the right path! If you always do the work of others, you are not a leader. You have not improved the situation. Knowledge is power and sharing knowledge is powerful. Giving yourself more work and spreading yourself super thin does not improve the workplace when others are in place for that purpose.

Taking responsibility is important. You will not only deal with sensitive information but also sensitive situations. If you make a mistake, be honest and take the proper steps to fix it. Sometimes your employer has those steps laid out in a policy or manual. If not, you need to notify your manager immediately and keep a record of what happened and what you did to resolve it. If you put up the wrong chart, scanned a document to the wrong patient account, credited the wrong account for a payment, handed someone the wrong script or order with another patient's name on it, these things must be addressed right away to reduce the liability of yourself and your medical facility and to protect your patients.

Responsibility also comes in the form of extensive call outs, tardiness, and lack of focus. You must be present to effectively perform your job and be a team player. Yes, everyone is entitled to time away from work, but when you work for someone else, there are rules and procedures that you must follow. That brings us to another important topic—Human Resources.

HUMAN RESOURCES

Human Resources is the division of a company that is focused on activities relating to employees. These activities normally include recruiting and hiring of new employees, orientation and training of current employees, employee benefits, and retention.[4]

The Human Resources department of your organization may be one person or a team of people who perform personnel-related functions. Why is this department important to you? This is the department that will assist you during your application and recruitment process. They also provide information on benefits, personnel policies and procedures. In many cases they handle payroll and time off requests as well. Before accepting any position, you should ask them all of the questions you have related to your benefit options, vacation and sick time, disciplinary actions, and training.

In my experience, employees tend to underutilize the expertise of the HR department. Once hired, they are

---

[4] http://www.businessdictionary.com/definition/human-resources.html

accessible, and you have every right to confirm policies and procedures, request assistance with interoffice issues and concerns, and discuss wage and salary issues. It is in your best interest to request a meeting, if needed. You should always be clear on what you have accepted as an employee, how your accrual of time works, what holidays are paid and which are not. All healthcare organizations are not the same. Just because your last position offered nine paid holidays does not mean the other won't only offer six! As I stated previously, read the employee handbook. Be educated. Stay in the light, not in the dark, when it comes to your time and money.

HIPAA, MOBILE DEVICES, AND EMERGENCIES

While I would love to dive into the deep formalities of private health information and privacy in general, I prefer to cover some of the more prevalent issues that front desk and medical clerical staff are usually faced with. How many times have you pulled out your phone at your station or have been working with a chart or patient documents and are called away from your station. In these quick instances, there are many things that can happen or be assumed. That is why it is your job to be cautious, aware, and protective of your patients' information as if it was your own.

If you leave a registration form face up on a desk and someone else walks right up, they can now see someone's name, address, social security number and other information that your organization requests. While most people would not look at it long enough to use it in a fraudulent way, they still see it. They then sit down and fill out the same form and hope that their paperwork is guarded more professionally. Since there is no one face for criminals, you cannot assume that all your patients will just have a seat! Aside from criminal acts, they may just take a picture to prove that you have been negligent and report it. These types of "mistakes" can cause a lot of damage to a medical group and parties involved. Lawsuits, reputation, identity theft, financial strain—you name it.

You may wonder why taking out your phone is a big deal. Let's move away from registration forms and consider that you are collecting payments. You have a patient's credit card, and while it's processing you decide to check a text message. The patient or others nearby can *assume* you took a picture of the card for later use. You could never prove that you didn't, unless there was a camera set up behind you. "Oh, I can just show the manager my phone." Guess what, I can take a picture, send it elsewhere and delete the immediate evidence. Why ever put yourself in a position for someone to even think that you could have done something like that? Instead, use your phone during breaks or request to step away from your station. Whatever you do, follow the rules of your employer. They are in place for a reason.

Stay focused. Don't leave records on the copy and fax machine for prolonged periods of time. Verify patients on the phone to ensure you are speaking to the correct party. Turn papers over when you walk away or take them with you until you have completed the data entry or filing. Be a team player; if your colleague has left medical records or other sensitive information out, turn it over and make sure it is not exposed to other clients. When you work as a team, every man or woman is not for themselves. It is everyone's job to protect the patient.

Talking is an easy way to violate the privacy of a patient. Never assume people don't know who you are talking about. If you are in a hallway or out in public going over stories from work, think twice. If you say too much you may reveal an identity to a third party without your knowledge. Imagine a friend telling you they overheard your current "status" at the local coffee shop, or they had an appointment at the office you both go to and the nurse and receptionist were talking about you in the hallway! You would be furious.

Let me tell you a few stories to bring this all together.

A patient once came into the office, signed in and asked to immediately be placed in a room because she saw a name of a person she knew on the sign-in sheet. While that is not a HIPAA violation, just that minor information altered how she felt about being in the office at the very moment.

What could have gone wrong? Perhaps a casual conversation between medical receptionists about the next patient, taking place in front of the patient who already signed in.

An employee allegedly confided in a friend on multiple instances regarding other patients in the office—people that they may have known locally. Eventually, the longtime friendship ended. Guess who reported violations against the office and used specific examples to attempt to harm her former friend's credibility and the practices of the organization? The "friend."

When it comes to the privacy of patients, it is not your place to share this information. Within the walls of the office only discuss what is necessary to provide the patient with quality care. Period. No excuses.

One day a patient came into the office, paid the copay, had a visit, and left the office. Within 24 hours he called the office because his credit card was charged for multiple online purchases. He did not contact the office to inquire; he came to accuse a staff member of wrongdoing. Why? Because that was the last place he had used the card.

When policies are loosely followed and phones are all over the desks, it is easy for someone to speculate the intentions of others when something terrible happens to them. Be mindful, make quick transactions, and return the card while the patient can see what you are doing, whenever possible.

A patient checks out and is handed her order for testing. She goes home and then calls the office and informs the staff that she was also given the order of another patient. These orders contain test and diagnosis information, patient information, as well as insurance information at times. She was kind and had called to notify and to make sure the other patient received what she/he needed and asked if it should be returned or shredded.

Imagine how many people won't call back. How many people would toss it, not shred it. Therefore, your attention is required during transactions. Moving fast to get your patients on their way is fantastic, but make sure you take the time needed to reduce errors and violations.

Let's dive into emergency procedures. Depending on the type of medical practice, facility, or hospital you work with, you should have been provided a very clear emergency plan and procedure. What kinds of emergencies happen in healthcare? All kinds. You may have a very ill patient decline in front of you; you may have someone experience a mental health issue which can no longer be contained in the office. There may be a toaster fire in the breakroom, bathroom flooding, power outages. Anything can happen. If you work within a specialty your exposure may be higher for a specific type of emergency. Whatever the case, you must take the procedures seriously. Know when to call "911," and know where the exits are. Get Basic Life Support (BLS) certified. If your employer does not offer this to you, inquire or obtain it on your own. Know what to do when police and EMTs arrive. Are you able to provide a patient's medical history? Did you inform a member of the clinical staff that can do so? When you called for emergency services, were you able to provide clear instructions for them to access your suite or floor?

How prepared are you?

Have you read the emergency policy from your employer? YES NO

Do you know where emergency equipment is located? (first aid kit, flash light, batteries) YES NO

Do you know where the wheelchairs are stored?
YES   NO

Can you quickly access a patient's emergency contact?
YES NO

Do you know how to perform the Heimlich maneuver?
YES   NO

Do you know what the active shooter protocol is for your office?   YES   NO

These are just some of the questions I want you to ask yourself in your current position and in the future. While I hope you never encounter adverse situations, in healthcare we have already signed up for a wild ride!

Most Required Skills—Let's Talk Job Descriptions

Greeting Patients and Visitors

Acknowledging patients, clients, and their families upon entry is usually the initial introduction to the physical space of the practice or organization. Welcoming words, attention, and a smile are usually enough to consider this a job well done. If your practice doesn't have a specific script, create your own. Have a longer version and a shorter version for really busy times. Actions such as this provide a consistent practice for you; you are also setting the bar of what good service looks like for your group.

Examples (Long) "Good Morning, I'm Alicia, welcome to Wood Rose Orthopedics. How are you today?" (wait for answer). "Have you been here before?" (wait for answer). "Great, please sign in, have a seat, and one us will be with you shortly,"

Example (Short) "Good Morning, I'm Alicia. Welcome to Wood Rose Orthopedics. Please sign in and we will be with you shortly."

Phones

This is one of the most important tasks completed by clerical employees. Whether you are answering direct lines, operating a switchboard or manning the various voicemail boxes and returning calls, you must be knowledgeable, courteous, a great communicator, and possess the ability to summarize and relay information in an effective and efficient manner.

Taking messages

It is not the length that is important. The accuracy and clarity of the message is key. If you find that your caller is not being specific enough, have a few questions that will get the information you know the doctor, nurse, or manager will need the answer to. For example, what symptoms are you experiencing? When did this start? Have you used any over-the-counter treatments? How long have you had the pain? When was the last time we refilled your prescription? Where would you like the letter sent?

Depending on the nature of your practice, develop a short list of questions that will be appropriate and also save time during the call. Correct spelling of names, dates of birth, and phone number are also key, not only for messages but for privacy and protection of the patient. If the patient is not willing to volunteer any information at least they can be identified and assisted by clinical staff or management.

What questions will you ask patients to improve efficiency?

_____

_____

_____

_____

_____

_____

_____

_____

Check in/Check out

Checking patient's in and out is the welcome and farewell of a medical visit. Check in, or registration, will generally include all or some of the following: signing in, updating insurance, scanning of insurance and ID cards, collecting a copy of records, collecting payments (copays/deductibles/balances), and placing the patient in que for the clinical staff. This task requires good customer service skills and organization. You want to make sure everyone who arrives is appropriately checked in and out. You want to make sure you received all the information needed when they arrive and that the patient leaves with any information that they need.

Insurance Verification

Insurance verification allows you to confirm that your patient has a current and active medical insurance policy. This can now be done in various ways. Some Electronic Medical Record or Practice Management systems can run an eligibility check once you have entered the information into the patient demographics. You can obtain this information via the insurance company's website or via a website such as Navinet, which allows access to multiple insurance carriers. You can also call the insurance company and obtain this information over the phone. Your facility will usually have a primary way of completing this task, but having access to multiple sources will come in handy when one resource is not available.

Demographics

Entering patient demographic requires you first obtain the information in writing and transfer the information to your computer system. Your accuracy on this task is very important. You will enter names, name changes, address, guarantor information, insurance, date of birth, emergency contacts and more. If your office is completely electronic, the patient may be entering most, if not all, of this information on their own. If this is the case, you must review for any inconsistences and make sure it has been completed in its entirety. If a patient's information is not entered correctly this can cause discrepancies with labs if the name is spelled wrong, reduction in collections if the mailing address is wrong and the patient is not receiving their bills, or even communication delays if they are not getting notices in the mail. In recent years a valid email address has become extremely important for general communication or portal notices. Never hesitate to ask someone for clarification if you cannot clearly read their writing. It will save a lot of time and headache in the future. The goal should be to get it right the FIRST time.

Payment Collection

Once you become familiar with the practice or facility payment collection policies you need to follow through with every patient. If you are only collecting copays, collect the copays! If you have the responsibility to collect co-insurance payments, deductibles, or old balances, you must be direct with the patient and question them every time. Consistency is key. If you mention that someone has a balance and they are unable to pay, you should be documenting and keeping note that you made the request. Don't stop asking because "they never pay." Your billing department or management will handle those overdue balances, but if the patient is still walking through the door for care it is your responsibility to make them aware and request payment on the account. If you do not understand the financial expectations, you must get familiar with the policies and process of your employer so you feel confident when discussing finances with your patients. There will always be certain cases that require a different level of intervention, but for your everyday transactions you must be prepared to do your part.

Scheduling

Scheduling appointments for checkup, procedures, injections, imaging, follow up exams and the like require you to follow the policies and timing set forth by your employer. Many offices have specified time frames for certain appointment types. Your practice may go a step further and require certain visit types not run back-to-back or they limit how many of a certain procedure they can perform in a day. This is done to make sure that all patients receive the time and care they need while in the office. It helps reduce patient wait times and provider burnout. Some offices run very smoothly with these methods. Other offices suffer due to acceptance of walk-ins and emergency or complex patient needs.

Managing Patient Flow

In healthcare we learn that things will not always go as planned. When the schedule is overloaded, or delays occur outside of your control, your job is to keep patients notified with updates and pay attention to the schedule as the day progresses. You may have to make calls and rearrange some appointments. The most important thing you can do in these situations is to keep the patients in the waiting room informed. If you know a provider is behind when a patient signs in, let them know immediately. This will reduce people coming up to the desk or becoming agitated after sitting, uniformed, for 40 minutes in the waiting room. If the appointment is not urgent some people may opt to reschedule because they have another appointment or conflict in their own schedule. Giving them the option to do this before they get all settled in is helpful. Providing delay notifications is a courtesy and shows that your practice also understands that your patient's/client's time is also valuable.

"I apologize for today's delay; we will call you in as soon as the doctor is available. Thank you for your patience."

Scanning/Faxing/Copying

These are basic functions that are required with any reception or clerical position. You must know the basic functions of office equipment. Some offices have machine that can perform these functions all in the one machine. Other offices may have a separate machine for each function. You will find with all the technological advancement, many of these products are networked with your work computer, allowing you to send, print, and fax directly from a patient's chart or your desktop.

Make it a habit to pick up any loose documents and don't leave patients information unattended for long periods of time on a machine. Complete the task and return the paperwork to the chart, the patient, or clinical provider. Whatever is not needed must be placed in designated shred bins or shredders. Don't let years go by before you learn how to make a double-sided copy. Initially, learn what you need to know, and when and if there is down time, look at the instruction manual. You may find out that the copier staples or can store documents that you use and copy daily. If you are making copies of a document that has been copied ten times before and it no longer looks crisp, find a good copy or create a new one that represents the office professionally.

Email

You may or may not be assigned a work email address. Since we have moved into a more digital age, employers want to be able to reach their employees with staff updates, insurance information, and company-wide notices, available trainings, and perhaps closings or delayed openings. If you are not an employee who receives many emails it is easy to leave your email account unopened for weeks and months on end. Make it a habit to check at least once a week or otherwise specified by your employer. Email is not a one-way street. It is also a way for you to communicate with your colleagues, management team, HR, and in some cases, patients. The email account is provided to you by your organization and you should follow the email and internet policies that are in place.

Confirmation/Cancelation Calls

Confirmation calls are appointment reminders via phone. If you are responsible for confirmation calls be sure to provide the patient date, time, and location (if you have multiple offices). Have a standard script so you can complete the calls efficiently. Tailor it to best suit your practice. If the patient needs to bring something with them that you are aware of—such as new patient demographics or a picture ID—mention it.

"Hi, Mr. Payne. I am calling to confirm your appointment with Dr. Rose tomorrow in our West office, December 30th at 4 pm. Please bring your insurance card, picture ID and copay. Have a great day!"

Pre-certification

Many health insurance plans require that pre-certification/prior authorization is obtained before a practitioner can perform certain procedures, provide medications, or medical equipment. The basic concept is that the insurance company wants to make sure that whatever a patient is offered is medically necessary and eligible for coverage based on the plan's guidelines. While an authorization is not a guarantee of payment it is always in the best interest of the office or facility to obtain one when indicated by a patient's insurance plan. Years ago, authorization was not as widely required as it is today, especially when it comes to medications and in-office services.

You may or may not have the responsibility of initiating prior authorizations within the practice. If you do, always make sure you know all the ways to obtain or initiate one—by phone, online portal, insurance site, or fax. These options will require you to have key information handy—basic demographics, service or medication, and exactly why it is being ordered. Therefore, you will not only need the name but the codes CPT and ICD. You will also need to know whether it will be completed inpatient or outpatient and the facility information, address, tax id, provider NPI. The more prepared you are, the smoother the process. Some insurance companies will require a copy of the patient's medical record or a conversation with a clinical provider. After a while you will see what process works best for different scenarios. Some procedures will be authorized immediately while others will require a few business days.

Computer/Internet/Microsoft Office

The general use of computers and the internet has become a basic skill in the healthcare industry. As technology advanced everyone had to get on board whether they had been in the field for two years or thirty-five years. You will often find that job descriptions will have Microsoft Word or Microsoft Office listed. The employer wants to make sure you can find your way around a Word document or Excel spreadsheet. If the position requires more than basic knowledge it is usually specified as an expert or advanced skill. Otherwise, you will find that performing the same functions on the job will allow you to learn quickly if you are a novice.

ICD and CPT coding/Medical Terminology

Diagnosis codes and Procedure codes are how a patient's visit is described in a numerical or alpha-numerical way. Mostly utilized for billing and claim purposes, every diagnosis has a corresponding ICD code and every procedure or visit type has a CPT code. Medical terminology is not always a required skill for a receptionist. However, if you are working in a medical setting you should at least obtain some basic information. You can start with terms directly related to your facility or specialty. If you are working within a multi-specialty group, you may never know what everything means but do your best to learn and use your resources, online or terminology and coding books. Most offices have them readily available.

BLS Certification

Basic Life Support or similar certifications are standard for clinical staff. It is now being more often recognized as a standard requirement for clerical staff as well. Medical facilities are finding it beneficial to have all staff certified. If promotes a level of quality and shows dedication to the safety of patients and staff. If an emergency were to arise, all staff could assist if absolutely needed. This is very helpful when you only have seconds to respond to a life-threatening emergency.

Reliable Transportation

When you are seeking new or initial employment as a Medical Receptionist always consider location and distance. If you have personal transportation, great. If you are relying on public transportation or a car service, weigh all of the options before accepting a position that is either too far away, too costly, or where you have an increased chance of missing many days of work due to weather, finances, or even the hours. Your employers' concern is not how you get to work; it is knowing that you CAN get to work when you are scheduled to be there. Many offices open very early and close in the evening. If you are gainfully employed and have never had an issue with transportation, keep a back-up plan that will be there if you ever need it.

ORGANIZATIONAL CULTURE

The values and behaviors that contribute to the unique social and psychological environment of an organization.[5] Organizational culture includes an organization's expectations, experiences, philosophy, and values that hold it together, and is expressed in its self-image, inner workings, interactions with the outside world, and future expectations. It is based on shared attitudes, beliefs, customs, and written and unwritten rules that have been developed over time and are considered valid. Organizational culture is also called corporate culture.

Many people tend to fall in line with the corporate culture, or rather, feel forced in line. If you understand more about the company you work for, it becomes easier to understand why they do what they do and why it may be different from anything you have ever experienced. Different is fine! New experiences are fine, too! It is important to know the mission of the practice,

---

[5] http://www.businessdictionary.com/definition/organizational-culture.html

hospital, or healthcare facility. Is it in line with what you experience in the office daily? Do you feel it resonates well with your own beliefs about work, community, patient care and quality, respect and responsibility? I sure hope so! If it does not, don't feel discouraged; feel empowered to understand before you decide that it doesn't work for you. Ask questions, be a part of the team and embrace the learning experience.

Every healthcare or medical facility has its own culture. The culture not only encompasses the career, professional, and quality of service provided. It also encompasses some fun stuff. Perhaps they celebrate all the time—birthdays, holidays, retirements—you name it. Everyone brings in their favorite dish or maybe the office treats lunch. Many people can connect more personally with their colleagues, learn their interest and share some laughs when these occurrences happen. That's great.

Not interested? If you have no interest in connecting or participating, be upfront and honest. It doesn't matter the reason, just be cordial about it. "I understand there is going to be a grab bag of gifts; I just prefer not to participate. Thank you for thinking of me." Done! You do not owe anyone anything. Whether you don't celebrate holidays, prefer to keep your money in your pocket instead of tossing it in that birthday pot, or do not wish to mingle outside of work, it is okay to say no and it is also okay for people to move on and not judge you for it. Period. The same with gossip. You can say, "No, not interested"! We have choices.

What if the culture changes over time? If you have been with the same employer for some time you may have witnessed co-workers, physicians, and managers come and go. While the core culture remains the same, the more "fun" activities may decrease or increase.

Many organizations have great employee recognition programs, team-building events, volunteer opportunities and more. Someone must spearhead those things. When you lose people who enjoyed creating, organizing, participating, and sharing in these experiences, some of what you used to look forward to goes away. This may also result in decreased morale, which then affects the overall culture and feel of the organization. Recognize when this happens and perhaps you can be the voice to bring that life back into the office. Don't assume that nobody cares. You are busy, your management is busy, HR is busy. Perhaps it just slipped their mind, or they figured since nobody has inquired they would just let it die. Don't forget, you are the bridge.

EMPLOYEE EVALUATION

Did you read the heading and see dollar signs? Healthcare, like any other field evaluates employees based on performance. The evaluation may be more general in nature and only become detailed when you have done something extraordinary or terrible. Evaluations can also be very specific to your daily duties, customer service, and communication.

How often should you be evaluated? Your employer should have a standard for evaluation of employees, perhaps 30-90 days after your initial start and then once a year. That is not uncommon. The information may be provided in your employee handbook. Your Human Resources department may also be able to explain the process. Just because you are being evaluated does not mean you are getting a rate increase. Remember, this is letting you know how you are doing, what you are doing well, where you can improve, and how the organization will help you meet any new goals.

While you may not get an increase at the time of the evaluation, when there is an hourly or salary increase it will most likely be partly based on your evaluation. What if you have not received an evaluation in years but have received reasonable rate increases over time? Good for you! However, you may want to know how you are really doing in the eyes of your manager or administrator. This will allow you to know where you stand and how you can make improvements or just continue the current path because you do awesome work! Request an evaluation. You need a record of your efforts. It pays to know; work is not necessarily the best place for surprises to creep up on you.

MONEY, MONEY, MONEY

Time to get green! Have you ever said the following? "They don't pay me enough to do that." "If I made more money I would be happier." "I need a raise." "My friend down the street is making more money." Well, let me start by saying, don't equate your paycheck with your happiness—we can discuss that in another book. However, you do have to live and provide for yourself and your family.

While people in all industries wake up feeling like they can be more heartily compensated, have you bothered to look at the industry standard for your area, your industry, or your experience level? You cannot just expect that you will be paid the amount you want. You can, but you may have to attain more education, experience and change careers. While you are at this point in your career, find out what makes sense for you right now, exactly where you are. If you have facts in hand you can then bring a valuable conversation to your employer if needed. They will respect your research and your professionalism. Walking into your manager's office and telling them that you couldn't make your car note or pay your mortgage is not truly their concern. That is not how a business determines wage increase. If everyone played the victim and was rewarded most organizations would not be able to handle the financial pressure. Just as you are not able to make everyone happy, neither can your employer. They can do their best by keeping wages competitive and even throwing in a bonus here and there!

Medical Receptionist Wage Tips:

- Do not use your coworkers' pay as an argument to increase your own

- Ask for what you believe you deserve, and have facts and outcomes to support it

- Do your research and understand the industry and specialty wages related to your area of the country

- Approach the situation with a positive attitude and a clear request

- Be prepared for a negotiation; don't be surprised if they turn down your initial request

- When you set a meeting to discuss a wage increase, make sure you let your manager or HR know why you want to meet. Let them be just as prepared as you are. If they ask to talk about it on the spot, let them know you prefer to speak during your scheduled time.

- What if you get a big fat NO?

  - ✓ Have a plan—do you want to stay and revisit in a few months?
  - ✓ Do you feel the position will no longer be a good fit at the current rate and plan to leave as soon as you can fulfill your personal needs?
  - ✓ Perhaps you were asked to wait until a specific time of year—will you wait?
  - ✓ If you feel the reasoning to be completely justified, do you just leave it alone all together?

Here are some resources to assist you.

- Bureau of Labor Statistics
  www.bls.gov Occupational Employment Statistics for Medical Secretaries

- Payscale www.payscale.com
  Medical Receptionist Salary

- Glassdoor www.glassdoor.com
  Unit Secretary Salary

TIPS AND REMINDERS

- Stellar customer service is key

- Introduce yourself, especially to new patients and new colleagues

- You chose to accept the position—get the job done

- Address issues and conflict professionally and immediately

- Gossip equals negative energy; it spreads like an untreated infection

- Be a team player—no practice or hospital stands on the shoulders of one person

- Patients are the priority and they should receive the quality of care your organization promotes

- Be respectful and be respected

- You are the bridge; your position and contribution are valuable

FINAL THOUGHTS

The Medical Receptionist Network Handbook was created to highlight some of the most important tools a Medical Receptionist can have: good and effective communication, accountability, organization, and professionalism. Also important is being resourceful and understanding with patients, co-workers, and management and taking a specific stance in your role as a medical receptionist, medical secretary, or unit secretary. One must understand the importance of the role they are in to truly be an asset. Your value to an employer is in your attitude, your willingness to learn, your ability to adapt, and your drive to succeed. Healthcare careers come in many forms—it's a huge industry! You may or may not have a college education; you may or may not have a lengthy background as a receptionist. That does not mean you cannot be the best at what you have chosen to do. You can become a part of the industry and embrace all of the learning experiences, education, training, constructive criticism, advice, and mentorship that is available to you.

ABOUT THE AUTHOR

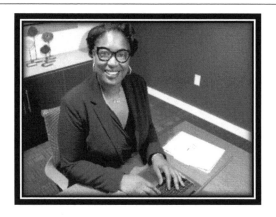

Shivhon is the founder of Medical Receptionist Network LLC. Shivhon has over 15 years of experience in the field of healthcare. She is also the Operations Manager of the Comfort Killers LLC, which specializes in Personal Development and Entrepreneurship. Shivhon is also the Owner of Love and Burn, an online retailer of soap and skincare products.

Shivhon earned her Master of Public Administration with a concentration in Health Services Management from Keller Graduate School of Management. She is an active member of The Professional Association of Health Care Office Management (PAHCOM).

Shivhon enjoys spending time with family, traveling and exploring new opportunities. Originally from New Jersey, Shivhon currently resides in Philadelphia, PA.